MY JOURNEY WITH HERBS

A personal journey of natural healing and faith

By Vivian Moody Perry

Disclaimer: I am not a medical doctor and do not claim to be one. I never took conventional medical courses, but I am a Certified Naturalist Consultant. I have studied with one of the world's renowned holistic naturalist doctor in the country. I have also taken courses with the Certified Natural Health Professionals.

Information on the traditional uses and properties of herbs provided in this book is for **educational use only**, and is not intended as medical advice. Many traditional uses and properties of herbs have not been validated by the Federal Drug Administration. If you have any serious health concerns, you should always check with your health care practitioner before self-administering herbs.

The information presented here is meant for educational purpose only and not as a substitute for medical treatment or diagnosis treat, cure or prevent any disease.

Understand that you are solely responsible for the way this information is perceived and utilized, and do so at your own risk. In no way will we be responsible for any kind of injuries or health problems that might occur due to the use of this book or the advice contained in it.

ISBN-13: 978-1477401668
ISBN-10:1477401660

TABLE OF CONTENTS
Introduction
Acknowledgments

My Story

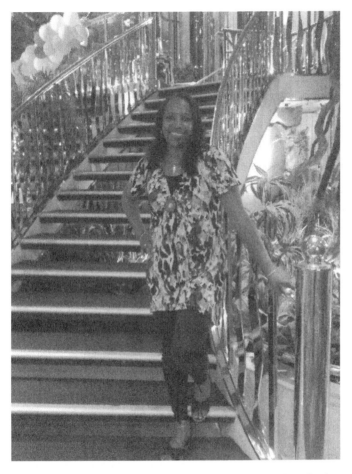

Photo taken: February 22, 2011, on the Norwegian Cruise ship, celebrating my big 60th birthday.

My name is Vivian Moody Perry. I am 60 years old and feel like I am 25. From a young age I have always had a passion to help people. I would ask God to please give me the gift to heal people. After watching my dad suffer from heart trouble, I wanted to be a healer of people. My dad would walk the floor at night moaning and groaning because of the excruciating stomach pain he had. As a child I would hear him moaning. I loved my dad so much that I would ask God to give me his pain for a minute. I just wanted my dad to have some peace if only for a minute. I knew I would not be able to handle such pain. However, when you truly love someone, we make difficult sacrifices. Jesus (Yeshua) made the ultimate sacrifice for us by going to the cross for our sins and healing.

I studied God's natural healing plants (herbs). I personally used the natural herbs to heal myself. I have not used conventional medicine for many years. I do not catch colds and have never had the flu until I took the flu shot. Twice I took the flu shots and both times I was sick for a week. After those two incidents, I have never had another flu shot; and that has been over 25 years ago. However, I have had some ailments which doctors claimed I was most likely born with.

After finding out my minor and major medical issues, I used various natural plants and I am completely healed from those diseases. I have never called these conditions a disease. I call it a temporary "dis ease." I must warn you of the one disadvantage herbs have, and that is, since it is all natural without chemicals it takes a little longer to heal than conventional medicine. However, everyone is different and some may heal faster than others. If I had a choice, I would take natural herbs any day compared to conventional medicine with its many horrific side affects.

I am not telling you what I have heard or read; I am giving you **first hand experience. I am a living testimony** of what God's natural healing plants can do.

If you read my story you will find out about all of the diseases that I have endured, and how through God's natural healing plants (herbs) I was healed.

This book is dedicated to my mother,
Lizzie Moody, a strong loving and wonderful Godly woman.
She taught us to strive for the best.

In Loving Memory of
My late father,
Vincent Moody a true Godly man who taught his children to
love the Lord.   I know he is with the Father in heaven.

Acknowledgments

First and foremost, I thank God for his Son, mercy, love and herbs.

Also, I would like to take this time to acknowledge and thank those who helped me put this book together. I would like to thank El and Pamela Harriatt, Founders of Merchants of the World, LLC, located at website: **www.Merchantsoftheworldstore.com**

They saw something in me which I did not know was there. They encouraged me to tell my story because God used me as a living testimony.

I would also like to thank Curt Worrell for his coaching, time and energy to help me put it all together. I want to thank my editor Ashley Brinkley.

Last but not least, I would like to thank my husband, Conrad Perry, and daughter, Melody Perry for being patient with me through this journey. Also, I want to thank my siblings for their encouragement and prayers. I could not have done it without them.

Much Love!

Chapter 1
First Encounter with herbs

I started dabbling and experimenting with herbs when I was in my early 20s. I read a few books on herbs and their miracle properties, one of the books was called "**Back to Eden**" by Jethro Kloss. My curiosity was peaked and from then on I wanted to learn more about the different herbs. To my surprise I found it very interesting learning about God's natural healing process through plants.

I remember my first time using herbs. It was a tea called *Bayberry Bark* and it tasted like the bark of a tree. It was supposed to help with your appetite and cleanse your blood. Women could also use this as a natural way to cleanse their vaginal areas internally. I felt great drinking this tea and I continued to drink it for some time until I could no longer tolerate the taste anymore. The taste was very bad. To keep the natural flavor and benefits, I did not use sugar or any artificial sweeteners and it tasted horrible.

Chapter 2
Trouble with Uterine (Fibroids)

As I got older I started having problems with a tumor in my uterus, a fibroid. The sad part was I didn't realize I had a fibroid until I was actually 21 years old. I went to my GYN for my annual checkup, and while examining me, he nonchalantly said,

"Oh! By the way, you have a fibroid tumor."

Being in my early 20s he said to me,

"Do not worry; it is the size of a dime so if it does not bother you do not bother it."

That was the end of that conversation, but I never forgot how I felt when I heard the words fibroid tumor. All I heard was the word *tumor* and the only types of tumors that I knew about were cancerous tumors. I cried all the way home on the subway. I remember just crying and thinking I had cancer and this male doctor was so cold. He did not explain anything to me other than I had a fibroid tumor, and I was basically too young to worry about it. At the time, I was still living at home with my mother and siblings. My mother came in to ask me how the doctor's appointment went only to find me crying hysterically. I was devastated thinking about the cancerous tumor that I had.

She asked me,

"What is wrong," and I told her I was just told by my GYN that I have a tumor. I know she was stunned because she stood there and I guess she too did not know what a fibroid tumor was.

Her reaction was,

"Well crying will not help anything."

She walked out of the room; because she was too devastated to let me see her anguish. I remember my sister who is two years younger than me come in and sat down beside me. I could not stop thinking that I was going to die. Suddenly my sister puts her arms around me and says,

"Do not cry it is going to be okay, Vivian."

I will never forget that she was there to comfort me in one of my darkest moments. My sister telling me

"Do not cry it is going to be okay Vivian,"

made me feel a little better.

After the way my doctor approached me and failed to explain anything about fibroid tumors, I referred to my book *"Back to Eden."* I looked up diseases and I found out what a fibroid tumor was and the cause. It comes from certain foods that we eat with too much estrogen. As a result of this the female body will produce this type of tumor. All females are naturally born with estrogen. We can't have too much estrogen in our body otherwise it causes havoc on our systems. I realized that this was a serious problem. However, I did thank God, because it never really bothered me because of its very small size.

Going forward for a couple of years I did not have a problem with my fibroid, because it did not grow. When I look back on why I think it did not grow, is because I was still at home. My mother cooked dinners everyday so there was no fast food and I almost never ate out.

The only time I did eat out was at my job's cafeteria. I do remember what I ate everyday at lunchtime which was a tuna or turkey sandwich. I did not eat much chicken or other meat. I still did not have a problem with the fibroid; it continued to stay very small.

Chapter 3
What is a Uterine Fibroid Tumor?

Fibroid tumors are benign (non-cancerous) growths. They appear on the muscular wall of the uterus. They range in size from microscopic, to masses that fill the entire abdominal cavity. Fibroids consist of dense, fibrous tissue which are nourished and sustained by a series of blood vessels.

Fibroid tumors of the uterus are a modern-day plague of women. Tumor is a word describing a bump rather than naming a disease. The muscle fiber of the uterus weakens and develops a bump-like ballooning out, similar to a hemorrhoid or varicose vein. Fibroids can grow with or without a capsule. Inside the fibroid capsule, there can be rotten blood, trapped veins, arteries, cellular waste, and a mass of muscle or fluid pus. The tumor can be the size of a bean or as large as a grapefruit or fetus. It can have various shapes, such as flat, oval, spider web like, mushroom, needle like or even grow like a tree. Fibroids are usually benign and non-cancerous and some do not require surgery. They tend to shrink during menopause due to decreased estrogen production.

Symptoms of fibroids include bloating, heavy menstrual bleeding, infertility, pain during intercourse, frequent urination, a feeling of pressure or pain in the pelvic area and constipation. Fibroids can be treated with the permanent removal of the uterus, through a hysterectomy or by doing a focused ultrasound surgery to neutralize the fibroids. A myomectomy, which involves the surgical removal of the fibroids, also allows women to have children later on while reducing the pain and bleeding they experience. Also useful is the detoxification of the liver, which helps control the hormonal levels, thereby slowing down the growth of the fibroids.

Facts:

Fibroids affect 40% of all women in America and have a high rate of incidence among African Americans. There is a possible link between uterine fibroid tumors and estrogen production. Fibroids do not grow before puberty when the body is not producing estrogen. They can grow very quickly during pregnancy, or if you are using birth control pills when estrogen levels are high.

There are many natural remedies for fibroid tumors, such as natural food diets, herbs, exercise, colonics, dancing, massage, meditation, herbal cleansing baths and spiritual rituals.

A natural food diet is one free of synthetic estrogen found in cow's milk, meat and eggs, and free of foods that dehydrate tissue (uterine), such as white sugar, vinegar, alcohol, sodas, salt, bleached white flour, polished white rice and caffeine. Caffeine causes the uterus to develop fibroids by decreasing the blood flow to the uterus, which causes waste to accumulate fibroids. Fibroids are waste isolated in a bump form called a tumor.

Excess Estrogen

Estrogen and steroid hormones are added to non-organic fruits, vegetables, milk, eggs, dairy and meats which cause excess estrogen.

Excess Estrogen causes:

- PMS
- Bone Loss
- Early Andropause
- Loss of sex desire
- Early Menopause
- Arthritis
- Vaginal Dryness
- High Blood Pressure
- Diabetes
- Dry Skin
- Low Sperm Court
- Baldness
- Split ends on hair

- Prostate disease
- Weight, water and/or fat increase
- Premature ejaculation
  and/or dribbling of urine (both sexes)

Different Types of Fibroids:

Internal Bump types; these abnormal growths occur within the uterine wall as well as in the connective tissues, especially the fibrous. Some fibroids include amounts of muscular tissue growth of a pale fleshy color and do not feel like growths, but are more similar to an inflammation. Some women are not even aware of having them.

Subperitoneal Fibroids; When they are massive, they give a sense of bearing down in the abdominal area and the abdomen as well as constipation, painful and difficult urination, malnutrition (nutrients are delivered to and absorbed by the tumor) neuralgia (pain) of the lower extremities, back pain and shortness of breath.

Submucous Fibroids; These have the same symptoms as the below interstitial fibroids but with increased severity. In addition to the excessive hemorrhage and menstrual colic, they are characterized by severe leukorrhea (whitish vaginal

Discharge). The leukorrhea is caused by the bloating of the skin of the endometrium resulting in mucous secretion. The colic is the primary result of labor like muscle contractions by the uterus in its efforts to expect the stagnated (rotten) blood in the dilated (bloated) vessels and or may be the cause of irritation by submucous polypi (stem-like tumor).[1]

Interstitial Fluids;
-can cause forward or backward tilting of the cervix, uterus, etc.

-can cause menstruation pain

-the primary symptoms are menorrhagia, (excessive bleeding during pregnancy) and metrorrhagia (uterine hemorrhage between menstruations accompanied by severe pain.) The hemorrhaging for menstruation is caused by excessive dilation, which weakens the blood vessels of the uterine wall.[2]

[1] "African holistic Health" by Dr. Llaila O. Afrika (pg.421)
[2] "African holistic Health" by Dr. Llaila O. Afrika (pgs.422-423)

Chapter 4
Pregnancy and Fibroid

At the age of 29 I got pregnant. Low and behold the fibroid grew with the fetus at an alarming fast rate. The fibroid grew so fast, and my stomach was so big that people thought I was having twins, but I was only having one child. I had an extremely difficult pregnancy. Carrying my daughter was very difficult and it was very dangerous. I had to wear a special girdle because I had to control her movement. As the fetus, my daughter, was growing so was the fibroid. The baby and the fibroid were both vying for the same space and the fibroid was resting on my nerves. If she kicked the fibroid, it would hit nerves and the nerves would send excruciating paralyzing pain to the whole left side of my body.

During my third month of pregnancy is when the fibroid really grew. I had such horrible pain on my left side. I had no idea what was wrong, and I was taken to the hospital. In the emergency room the doctors had no idea what was wrong either. I would make weekly trips to the emergency room to figure out what the problem was. Most of the time my doctor was always on vacation. At the emergency room internal examinations were given to me, and all they would say was,

"The fetus is intact so we don't know what the problem is."

I never told them about the tumor because I did not think it was the culprit. I did not know it was growing due to my body producing extra estrogen from my pregnancy. I had no idea that the tumor would grow but it did. The doctors would send me home and I could barely walk because of the piercing intense pain. For a week straight my sister or another member in my family would take me to the emergency room. The doctors still could not figure out what the problem was. Since they did not know my medical history, they would just send me home. I would stay home, sit, cry and pace around the house. I was absolutely miserable those first six months of pregnancy. The pain was so bad that I never wanted to have another child. Just the thought of having another baby, and the pain that I went through carrying my daughter would make me cry. I only have one child and have only experienced pregnancy once. I know my doctor and everyone says each pregnancy is different, but I did not want to chance it.

When I got home, once the emergency staff said there is nothing they could do, finally my GYN returned from his vacation. I called him right away and over the phone I told him what happened, and how I had to go to the emergency for an hour. His reply to me was,

"Oh! you have a fibroid and it grew. The fibroid tumor grew and that's why you are having pain. The baby and the fibroid are fighting for the same space."

I was very upset with my doctor, I said,

"Well, why did you not tell me, you are my doctor, you're my GYN. You are my doctor why would you not tell me when I got pregnant there is a possibility the fibroid could grow."

His reply was,

"Well, yeah, there's a possibility but not every body that has a tumor grows. Your tumor just happened to be one that grew. You just have to get used to living with pain."

I got off the phone from him, and I said okay hopefully it will stop, but the pain never stopped. I went to my GYN again and told him I can't deal with this pain anymore, I want you to remove the tumor. He replied,

"I can't remove the fibroid because you are pregnant and there is no way I can do that. You would lose the baby."

Since I was in such excruciating pain, I told my doctor I wanted the baby out. I want to abort the baby I can't do this, I can't go another six months in this pain it is just unbearable. The doctor then said to me,

"Vivian, this is a serious matter, think about it, talk to your family and to the baby's father. This is something very serious here, think about it."

I talked to my daughter's father, who is now my husband, and I asked him what he thought. He told me,

"I can't tell you what to do, because I do not know how much pain you are in."

I spoke to my mother about it and told her what I wanted to do. I wanted to get rid of the baby and tumor because of the pain and I could not bear it for the next six months. My mother's response was,

"The baby is a blessing from God and do you really, really think that you want to do this?"

I then turned to my best girlfriend in the world. She is like a sister to me. I told her exactly what I wanted to do, how miserable I was and how I was always in pain. I didn't get the answer I was looking for, but she gave me the one that I am thankful for. She gave me a slap back to reality and she said to me,

"What did you think having children is easy? Yes, some people are lucky and there are some women that have it easy. The majority of women go through a lot to have their babies and it is painful. Once that child comes into the world it is all worth it. Stop being a wimp, she said, I have had two kids and I have had extremely difficult pregnancies where I had to stay on bed rest."

She continued,

"Vivian, it is not easy but, you can do this".

I did not have the abortion and went through with the pregnancy. I talked to God, searched my heart and thanked him for the pregnancy. It is a blessing to have a child. A blessing from God and I asked for forgiveness and to give me a normal pregnancy and a healthy child. From that day forth, as God is my witness, I can truly say I did not have any more excruciating pain like I had at the beginning.

Once I did what the doctors told me by wearing specialized underwear and a girdle, the pain got better. The baby movements were restricted and there were certain things I could not do. When I followed their instructions and believed that God had taken the pain away, I did not have the excruciating pain anymore. Every now and then I would get a little discomfort when she kicked but it was not like before. However, the fibroid kept growing with my daughter.

I delivered my child and I had a healthy eight pound two ounces beautiful daughter. I thank God and my best friend for bringing me back to reality about having a child. I told my daughter the story, and every time she sees my best friend she is grateful and says,

"I know because of Ronnie I am here."

My daughter is the best blessing I could ever imagine and we are best friends. I could not imagine a life without her.

Chapter 5
Fibroid After Delivery (birth)

Now getting back to the procedure of the fibroid. So the fibroid is huge, and now my doctor and I figured after having the baby that we're going to remove this fibroid. But amazingly after I had my baby, the fibroid shrunk to the size of a peanut. When I went back to my GYN, and during the internal examination my doctor noticed the fibroid tumor had gone down to the original size of a peanut. It was amazing that it would grow to be the size of the fetus and then go down to the size of a peanut. My estrogen level had decreased substantially after the birth making that the main reason why it decreased. It was a great feeling to have no more pain and swelling of the stomach. As the years went by I had no problem with my fibroid.

I pay attention to how my body reacts to what I eat. Also, when I do something different or take different pills I pay attention to how it affects my body. I know every little mark that is different that was not there before. I have always been that way and I teach my daughter to be the same way to know her body.

At this stage in my life, I have a new female Gynecologist (GYN). I feel that male GYN's do not really know a female's body. He does not go through what we do, monthly periods, mood swings, menopause and other female problems. Please do not misunderstand me, most male doctors are good, but they do not have a vagina and can't really relate to females. They go by the book and second hand knowledge. Whereas, a female GYN knows first hand what we are going through because she is a woman. I am very pleased and comfortable with my female GYN.

On my first visit to my new GYN she gave me an internal exam. She informed me I have fibroids and said they are small, and there is nothing to be concerned about. She tells me that my one fibroid has now turned into five. This is a couple years later as my daughter was now about six years old. I am now thinking how did they increase and where did they come from?

Chapter 6
Outrageous Growth of Fibroids

I was going away with my husband on a cruise, and I wanted to get my body in great shape. I wanted to look nice in my swimwear, and so I started a strict diet and exercise regimen. I distinctively remember everyday going out for lunch with my friend and getting the same meal. I would have a chicken sandwich, sprite soda with a pickle and potato chips. I know exactly the type of meal that I purchased because it was pretty good with honey mustard on the chicken sandwich. Everyday for the next three months I ate this for lunch. I was preparing three months in advance for my vacation.

I ate chicken for three months as I am getting ready for my vacation with my husband. However, I noticed a change in the second month on this new diet. I noticed that my periods are starting to get heavier. I am starting to bleed heavier and longer. Even though they are getting longer, I still don't think much about it. I am going through some changes in my body but did not pay much attention to it. I was only focusing on my much needed vacation.

I go on my vacation return home and I have my annual checkup with my GYN. My GYN gives me an internal examination and then all of a sudden she starts to yell at me.

" Vivian, what did you do?"

She is very stunned at what she feels in my uterus. I am nervous as to what she is talking about and why she is so upset. I asked her,

"What do you mean, what did I do?"

She said,

"Your fibroids have grown very large in such a short time. How could they grow that fast compared to last year? Last year you had five fibroids, that were the size of a walnut, but now they are the size of an orange."

"What did you do?"

"I don't know, I have done nothing."

She is really concerned because she said they grew too fast in such a short time. I could not figure out what was wrong. What could I have possibly done differently to get such drastic results?

As time went on I love my new figure because I have lost so much weight and I am looking great. I am still eating the same chicken sandwich at lunchtime. Everyday we go to the same restaurant; and one day I noticed that I can feel the fibroids. I could feel the bulge or hard mass in my stomach and my periods are heavier than ever.

Chapter 7
Hemorrhaging

Now it is almost to the point of where I am hemorrhaging and it is lasting longer than seven days. I still can't put my finger on what was happening. All I knew was that something is growing in my stomach. My sex life was being affected, it was very painful and I could not bear to have my husband touch me around my stomach area. Especially in the morning, my stomach was huge and there was so much pressure in my pelvic area. I always felt constant pressure on my bladder and constipation.

I go back to my GYN and I am telling her the new problems that I am having, and she says to me well, yeah, she said you are hemorrhaging.

"Vivian," she said, your fibroids are very large."

She sends me to the hospital only a block from her office to get a sonogram. They will take pictures and really see what size they are she informed me. A week later I return to my doctor's office for the results. I was not prepared for what she told me. I sat down with her and she said,

"You have five fibroids one the size of a six-month old fetus, the other four the size of small grapefruits. They are large and that is why your stomach is protruding and you look like you are pregnant. Vivian, I suggest you have a complete hysterectomy because you are hemorrhaging. If you do not, you are going to have a heart attack or stroke. You need to have this done right away. Since you are in your 40's, I am sure you do not want anymore kids and we are just going to give you a complete hysterectomy."

Devastation & Jubilation

I was just devastated when I heard about the complete hysterectomy. She is a great doctor; but the way she explained it was as if it was a minor procedure. You have a little cut and put a band aid on the cut. I felt it was more than just getting a cut and healing with a band aid. Taking all of my female organs out was not normal for me.

I told my doctor, "It is not natural. God did not give me this, man did. It is what we are eating. I do not know exactly which foods it is, but I know the food has to be the cause." She replied,

"Well, African-Americans, Indian women and Latino women for some reason seem to be cursed with these fibroids."

"I do not know if it has to do with any of our food. I think is just pigmentation that may have attributed to this."

I said,

"No, I don't believe that. Give me three months. If three months later, these fibroids are still this size and I am still hemorrhaging I will have the operation. Just give me three months."

"I believe in a higher being (God). I believe in the man upstairs and it is just not natural to have this operation. I will then have to take all types of medication to replace what I have now lost which you have taken away."

She replied,

"Okay three months."

In "**Back to Eden**" it makes reference to an herb called (*RED CLOVER*) that cures or shrinks tumors. In the interim, while I was doing this, I met a naturalist named El at a flea market in New Jersey. I talked to him about fibroids and all my health problems. I tried his fibroid product called (*Red Clover*) and my fibroids started to decrease. When I went back to my doctor the fibroids were gone, they had dissolved. This all happened within *three months*. I took the (*Red Clover*) herbs. I took *1 pill 3x a day for three months*. To this day I am fibroid free without a costly and painful operation. I used God's natural healing plants.

Yes, they dissolved within three months. It may sound like that is impossible but with faith and determination it became possible.

After the three months I returned to the doctor for my checkup. When she was giving me the internal exam, she could not feel anything. The fibroids where gone they seemed to have melted away. Since she did not operate on me, it did not make medical sense to her. She was baffled and she asked,

"Okay what did you do? What happened here?"
I replied,

"I believe in God's healing plants and I changed my diet, I started taking herbs (**Red Clover**) as my medicine."

She was curious to know what did I take, I told her and watched as she took notes.

"How did you change your diet?"

Well,

"First of all, most milk has growth hormones in it. They are pumping up cows and our meats with growth hormones to make them bigger, better and fatter. I was eating foods with estrogen and noticed the fibroids were growing. When I realized that, I stopped and I changed my diet.

I started eating organic meat, chicken and fish. I took red meats out of my diet. I just eat fish and chicken. My chicken has to be organic or all natural, because they are hormone free."

Note: I would like to say that I took 3 capsules a day, however, my body is much stronger than most women and I usually have to double up on any herbs that I take. Therefore, I suggest you start off taking 1 capsule a day. Since organic herbs are much stronger than regular herbs. Whenever you introduce anything new in your body, pay close attention to how your body reacts.

Suggested usage: *Before taking Red Clover capsules, we highly suggest to go to your physician and test your estrogen level. If your estrogen level is high, we do not recommend that you take Red Clover. If your estrogen level is low and you want to try Red Clover, then we suggest you take one capsule for 90 days and then test your estrogen level.*

Chapter 8
Final Sonogram to Verify The Results

My doctor lets me know she has to send me to the hospital to get a sonogram again. I am lying on the table and the technician is inside of me. She is examining me and says,

"Well, Ms. Moody, when did you have your operation?"

I replied, "I never had an operation."

She replies,

"No, Ms. Moody, I want to know when did you have your operation?"

I said, "I have never had an operation"

Now she begins to get irritated with me. She turns around puts her pen down, and says to me very sternly,

"Ms. Moody I am looking at your charts from last year. I am inside of you and I am looking at the screen, and last year you had five fibroids one the size of a six-month fetus. I am looking inside you now and you have only one the size of a dime, and you are telling me you didn't have an operation. That is not medically possible. Now I am going to ask you one more time, Ms. Moody, when did you have your operation?"

So at that point, I smiled and laughed and said, "Well, let me ask you something, do you believe in God?"

She said, "Yes, I do."

"Do you believe he has healing plants?"

She replies, "Yes, I do. I do believe in his herbs. What did you use if you did not have an operation?"

I said, "Well, I used a special herbal product called (*Red Clover*)."

After I gave her the name of the product, I told her how I used it and she wrote it down and replies,

"Oh! My goodness, thank you, thank you, where can I buy this?"

I realized that herbs (**Red Clover**) really work when you change your diet, eat right and do not put trash into your body. I was sold on it. I use herbs for just about everything and there are so many diseases that I have used herbs to cure them.

True healing or Placebo Test

Everyone may think I am crazy concerning what I did next. I wanted to make sure the foreign (anything not organic) chicken was the culprit of my fibroids. I deliberately resumed eating the foreign chicken and I stopped taking my **Red Clover**. I ate chicken everyday for a month, and within that month the fibroid started to grow again. Not only did it return, but it grew faster and larger. My husband was my unwilling witness to this. I had him place his hand on my stomach and fill the bulge again. He could not believe what he felt. Now to test my other theory and make sure the **Red Clover** actually shrinks the fibroid and it was not a placebo, I resumed taking my **Red Clover**. I doubled the dosage because I wanted to shrink the fibroid faster. Within one month the fibroid was gone again. My husband was so amazed that he now tells his male friends about **Red Clover** for their female family members.

Chapter 9
Diet Changes

I changed my diet and took the herbal medicine (**Red Clover**). I took one capsule three times a day for three months and within the three months they were gone.

My mother, my grandmother and my aunts have never had any problems with fibroid tumors. As a matter of fact they have never heard of them. They have never had any female problems. The reason is that my grandmother and her family where farmers from the south. They ate the food from the land. They did not use pesticides or hormones to fatten their meats. Their food was natural food straight from the land. It is just these last thirty years that women of all colors and races are having problems, especially if you are eating red meats. I investigated and spoke to my elders about what they ate during their younger years.

Scientists are now trying to get the FDA to allow them to give farm raised Salmon fish hormones to make them come to full growth faster. However, no test has been made to determine what the ramifications to humans would be. It is as if they are trying to push *Frankenstein* food on us.

Chapter 10
Carotid Arteries

Next is my journey with blocked carotid arteries in my neck. Let me explain what carotid arteries do. Carotid arteries are on the left and right side of your neck. We have two major arteries that lead up to your brain and there is one in the back of your neck that leads up to the brain. Of course, if either one of them is blocked there is a possibility that you could have a massive stroke and die; because the brain will not get blood functioning to the brain properly.

I went for my routine checkup and I would say I was about 45 or 46 years old and that may seem old to some but to me that is still young. I went for a routine check up by my general practitioner. He listened to my pulse on my neck with his stethoscope. My doctor continued to listen to the left side of my neck. He checked my heart again and then did an EKG. When he finished the examination he said to me,

"Vivian, something does not sound right in your carotid arteries. I want to send you to a cardiologist specialist just to check it out."

What pops into my head when I hear the word cardiologist is my dad who passed from heart problems and that really worried me. I was truly concerned because my dad died at a very young age of 40 years old from a severe heart attack.

Anyway my doctor sent me to an expert cardiologist. I went to the cardiologist; he took numerous tests, and just said,

"Vivian, by the sound of the way the blood is flowing trying to get to your brain I can tell that you have blockage in you arteries."

I was again devastated; I have blockage in my carotid arteries. I was speechless, carotid arteries I have a blockage is all I could think. So I think okay, yes I am young so it can't be that bad. I had to take numerous tests. Some were even specialized tests. As it turns out, my tests came back showing I had 70% blockage (left side) plaque and 20% blockage in my (right side) carotid arteries. Those are numbers I will never forget. My cardiologist explains to me,

"We can't operate to remove the blockage because this is a major operation and you are too young. So what we have to do is take precaution by using the prevention method."

I asked, "Prevention? How do you prevent this?"

"The way we prevent this is that you would have to go on medication for the rest of your life. You have to go on a medication called Plavix."

"You will also you have to go on blood pressure medication."

"Blood pressure!" I said, "But doctor I do not have high blood pressure, so why would you put me on medication if I do not have high blood pressure."

He replied,

"This is because we have to make sure your blood pressure never elevates or it could lead to a stroke. If your pressure elevates a piece of plaque could break off and travel to your brain, and that is why you have to go on high blood pressure medication."

I am very upset because I do not want to take blood pressure medication due to the side effects. I have heard the side effects of high blood pressure medication are dizziness, depression and many other side effects. I just did not want to take the conventional medication. My cardiologist says to me,

"Okay, if you have blocked carotid arteries you definitely have blocked heart vessels. We must take further tests to determine how much blockage is in the heart."

This test is called catheterization where they go into the groin area and they put a tube into the artery to shoot dye up into the heart to see how much blockage is in my heart. So I had the procedure done, because 90% of the times when you have that much blockage in your carotid arteries you are going to have blockage in your heart. The procedure was done while I was awake. I heard the doctors say,

"Oh! My goodness she has got a beautiful heart, there is absolutely nothing there, and her heart is just great."

I was elated that my heart is great, and they are talking "but how can that be? We have never met a patient like this; it just does not make medical sense. If she has that much blockage in her carotid arteries, she is supposed to have blockage in her heart. However, her heart is like a young heart, she has got a perfect heart."

I heard all of that while I was lying on the table in the lab. I turned my head to see my heart on the monitor screen. When I revisited my doctor, he says;

"Vivian, we have taken every test known to man, but every test has come back negative."

I took so many tests it was unbelievable trying to figure out what was wrong with me. Was it something in my blood, how can I have that much plaque to be so young, and there is none in my heart.

My cardiologist said to me,

"I have been practicing for many years, and I have never in all my years of practice met anyone else like you except one other girl, she was 17 years old and had the same problem. Her heart was clear also. You two are the types of patients that we do special reports on, because we have never come across anyone in the medical field who has had this. I do not know what to tell you.

My colleagues and I can't figure out why there is no plaque in the heart area. Why and how could you have this much plaque in your carotid arteries? You are healthy, your pressure is good, and your weight is good. There is nothing else wrong with you. I just can't figure it out Vivian. The only thing I can say is that you are a freak of nature,"

We laughed about it.

He implied,

"In all truth, you had to be born like this, because people 80 years old and older have this much plaque. Anyone under age 80 does not have that much plaque. It takes years for you to have this much plaque, and it is a slow process of accumulation. You had to be born with it. It had to be hereditary; your father may have had it as well. Since he died from having heart problems, he may have had plaque buildup."

However, my father was not born with heart trouble. He contracted rheumatic fever as a child and it left a hole in the valve of his heart.   Medical technology was not as advanced as they are now. My father had open-heart surgery and from that day on he deteriorated and died at the age of 40.

My cardiologist said,

"All we can do for you is put you on Plavix and high blood pressure medication. You have to watch your diet; you will always need to visit the cardiologist so he could check and make sure it is not increasing. I would like to do a report about your case, as it is so unique."

When I left the doctor's office I was depressed, because I had to worry about plaque breaking off. ʒain, I prayed thanked God and said,

"Well God, when you give me discomfort you do not just give me minor discomfort you give me something that is just outrageous. The same way you healed me with your natural herbs you will do it again, and I have faith and I am thanking you in advance.

I am going back to my natural herbs. I am not taking the doctor's medication. I am going to your natural herbs and trusting in you for my supernatural healing."

Again, I went back to my herbal book to read about plaque. I read that the best thing for plaque in the whole world is *garlic*, good old-fashioned *garlic* that is hard to believe, it is something so simple, something we love to eat. I started taking it; and I got into a regimen where I would take one *garlic* pill three times a day. One at breakfast, lunch and dinner but I did not take it with food; I took it with out food because I did not want it to repeat. I took so much garlic I smelled like walking *garlic.* I had *garlic* coming from every orifice of my body. I did that for four years straight non-stop. I was on a mission to have my body healed supernaturally through God and his healing plants.

Each year I would go to the doctor and the technician would say to me,

"It seems to be decreasing, however, that is weird."

When my cardiologist got the results from the technician, he too was amazed because the blockage seemed to be decreasing.

"I don't know Vivian this seems to be decreasing but that just can't be," he said.

My doctor just assumed it was a mistake made either by the machine or technician. Every year the plaque would decrease, and I remember in the third year he said to me,

"Wow! I do not know what it is you are doing, but it is decreasing."

I said, "Well, doctor the only thing I am doing is taking good old-fashioned garlic"

He started to laugh.

"*Garlic*, you think *garlic* is going to, help"

"It is helping," I replied.

My general practitioner told me the same thing about *garlic*,

"Oh! That's a joke Vivian, *garlic* is not going to help decrease your blockage or get rid of that problem you have."

I held strong and I had faith. I believed in Jesus (Yeshua), and in his healing plants and supernatural healing. The fourth year was the best time. I always make mental notes of my results. I make sure that I keep my dates accurate as to how long it takes for the problem to clear up. When I went back, in the fourth year, to my doctor he gave me additional tests. He was listening but he was not hearing anything alarming. The blood seemed to be flowing very well. It seemed to be flowing to my brain, no problem with either carotid artery. After that, I went to see the technician, who has been there for the past four years. She set me up for another echo sonogram. The test was completed in 20 minutes and when she finished and looked at the results,

She asked, "Why are you here?"

I said, "Because I have blockage in my carotid arteries, they told me I have 70/20."

She took a look at my test results that were printing from the machine,

and says, "I can't find anything."

I jumped off the bed and I started to say,

"Thank you Lord, thank you, thank you, thank you Jesus."

I am praising God. The technician said,

"Well, who is your doctor, he may have made a mistake."

"No, I said, my doctor is Dr. M."

She replied,

"Oh no, he does not make mistakes."

Now she is confused and doubting herself.

"My gosh!" she said, "Did I do the test incorrectly."

She then runs into the next room and retrieves my chart history for the past four years.

She said,

"You are right there was something here, but each year it seemed to decrease. Oh! My goodness." She said, "I didn't make a mistake, the machine didn't make a mistake, and it is gone. What did you do? I don't understand it, what did you do?"

I asked, "Well, do you believe in God?"

She said, "Yes."

"Do you believe he has natural healing plants?"
She replied,

"Of course I believe that, I am Russian and my family does not use these medicines. We use plants; my family goes out to the garden and gets herbs."

I reply,

"Well, guess what I took? Good old-fashioned 100% *garlic* capsules everyday for four years."

She remarked, "This is amazing."

The proof was in the test results and there was no way of denying it. The sonogram told the story. When I went into the office of my cardiologist and he read the report that it was gone, he could not believe it.

He said,

"I can't believe this; I can't believe it is actually gone. There is nothing there on both your left and your right that is amazing."

"Since that has never happened before and you never had an operation, your carotid arteries were probably twisted and that caused us to assume there was blockage."

My doctor could not and would not accept that I took only *garlic* for my cure. He was convinced that my arteries were twisted and they were now untwisted. He was only satisfied with a scientific reasoning for my twisted (blocked) arteries. However, my general practitioner said that arteries can't twist or bend, and that was a ridiculous statement from my cardiologist.

My cardiologist says,

"Well, I guess you do not have to come here anymore,"

I was so thankful to God that it was gone and I could not stop praising Jesus when I left the office. As I was walking out, the staff also heard me praising God. They were all smiling and clapping for me and it was a remarkable feeling. I realized from that moment on that God had a purpose for my life.

I said, "I see what you are doing God, you have given me these diseases and outrageous things because you are using me as a <u>living testimony</u>."

If you have **faith** and you trust in him and his Son, he can heal you. You do not have to use conventional medicine; you can use natural medicine with hardly any side effects. God wants us to turn to him for our every need, healing, comfort, financial worries whatever we need. He is our big daddy and he is here to take care of his children.

Garlic has many miracle properties, it is a blood thinner that cleanses your blood and gets rid of parasites. It does so much for your body and may be one of the best natural healing plants, in addition to making our food taste so good.

I believe that God wants everyone to know about his healing plants, and that you do not have to use conventional medicine only. You have another option (herbs). If you feed and treat your body like a temple it will heal thyself. A famous Doctor by the name of *Hippocrates* once quoted,

"Natural forces within us are the true healers of disease."

I agree with this quote. Let me just reiterate that everyone should go to his or her doctors and get their annual checkups. I know better and go to all my doctors, get my checkups, and get a clean bill of health. If something is wrong, then I take my herbal medicine.

That was my journey with the carotid arteries that were blocked 70/20 percent. Now that everything is clear, I watch my food. I try to stay away from foods with a lot of cholesterol.

Each time I go to my general practitioner he gives me a clean bill of health. Also, you have to exercise because what you do not use, you lose. The body was built for motion, and we must move our body with at least 30 minutes of exercise everyday.

Chapter 11
SINUS Problems

I have had so many problems with my body. I had a sinus problem at one point. I would get nauseous and very dizzy. I could barely walk straight, my nose was hurting, and I could not breathe and had a migraine headache. I did not know what was going on. All I knew is that at a certain time of year this would happen.

It was embarrassing every time I would eat anything hot my nose would suddenly start running without a warning. I did not realize then, that the heat was making the sinuses drain which was a good thing. This went on for some time and I decided to visit the doctor. They gave me a test and determined I had severe sinus problems. The sinus problem became very debilitating at some point.

One of my coworkers had a sinus operation. She had her sinuses removed, and said it was extremely painful. Other people also told me that you can have them removed but they can eventually grow back. Unfortunately, after three years my co-worker had sinus problems again.

I spoke to her about the possibility of having an operation. She told me not to do it because all the pain she went through and all the money she paid for this medical procedure was a waste of time. Her sinus problem recurred. Okay, now what do I do? I tried all the over-the-counter drugs they would help a little but not much.

One day, that I will never forget, I got up from my chair to go into my boss' office and, I was so dizzy that I actually walked right into her glass door. My equilibrium was off and I could not balance myself.

Everyone grasped and said, "Wow! What is wrong Viv?"

I replied, "I can't walk straight my head is in such pain"

My boss said,

"Why don't you go to the doctor at the New York Stock Exchange building, there are doctors on site."

The doctor from the NY Stock Exchange looked at my nose, my ears and he said, "You have to be absolutely miserable. Your sinuses are so large and how are you breathing. How could you stand it, you must be in a lot of pain."

I responded,

"I am."

He replied,

"Well, we need to drain them, those sacks have got to be drained as soon as possible."

He stuck something into my nostrils trying to make it drain. Unfortunately, they would not drain.

"They will not drain, he said."

I replied, "Yes, I know, that is the problem they will not drain."

He gave me some medication to help drain them, but it did not help them drain. Now I am beyond miserable. I repeatedly got sinus infections all the time. Most people get colds but I would get sinus infections.

One day I had a cold sore on my mouth and I asked a friend what is good for cold sores. What she told me changed my life.

My coworker said,

"*Tea Tree Oil* it is an herbal liquid."

I purchased the *Tea Tree Oil* from the local drugstore. I put a little Tea Tree Oil on a cotton ball and I put it on this huge cold sore that I had. The next morning it was completely gone. That was so unusual because usually when I have had cold sores in the past, they last for a couple of days; and then they blister up and look very nasty. This one was completely gone, it was nothing there and I was surprised. I proceed to read its medicinal purposes. I had never heard of *Tea Tree Oil*; to my amazement it is good for scalps, fungus, and for burns. It is good if you have sores in your mouth, and sinuses. Bingo! These were magic words, *"sinus problems."* If you have never smelled *Tea Tree Oil*, it has a very pungent smell. Some people say the smell really bothers them. I have gotten used to it and I put it on a cotton ball, with equal parts of water on the cotton ball in both nostrils. I did that everyday and by the end of day three, my nose had started to drain. The poison that was in my sinuses finally drained. It was draining so much that I literally had to keep a tissue to my nose as it was draining, but it felt so good that I could breathe again. I remember for a whole week I took that bottle of *Tea Tree Oil* with me everywhere. I took it to work and I would go into the ladies room to drain my nostrils. When I returned to my desk, my boss came out of her office and she asked,

"What is that smell?"

I answered,

"I am very sorry that it is offending you but I really, really need to use this."

I would do that all day for a week, and by the end of the week my sinuses were completely flat. All the poison in the sacks and infection was gone. I felt great that I did not have to think about sinuses anymore. I thought no more misery, no more cloudy headaches, and it was amazing. I was so thankful and happy that I decided to use the *Tea Tree Oil*. After going to all those doctors and taking all those tests, it still doesn't compare to the painful sinus removal operation I was considering. I was so thankful for the young lady who recommended *Tea Tree Oil*. I gave her a bouquet of flowers as a thank you. I told her she made a big difference in my life by having my sinuses drain naturally. I was absolutely miserable and all it took was something natural, and not the doctors' recommended medicines that did absolutely nothing. To this day I love *Tea Tree Oil*. I always keep a bottle of it in my purse in case I cut myself; get a scratch, a burn, mosquito bites or any other skin irritations. I immediately put *Tea Tree Oil* on it and the next day my wound is fine. I also keep a bottle or two in my home.

Once I was cooking on a George Foreman grill making a hotdog. I forgot and didn't realize that the outer pot was hot on the grill, and I thought I was lifting the top. However, I wasn't and my finger got stuck. It was so hot it seared my finger; but I was able to pull my finger away. There was a big mark and indent on my finger and it was burning. It hurt so badly I immediately reached in my purse and put *Tea Tree Oil* on my thumb. Everyone is saying,

"Well you are going to have a huge blister tomorrow, and it is going to be painful. That is a nasty looking big burn straight across your thumb."

After putting *Tea Tree Oil* on it within an hour the burning completely stopped. The next morning, everyone knew that I was going to have this big blister on my finger. I showed them the spot where the blister was, and there was nothing there. It was a pretty pink thumb, there was nothing there everyone thought it was unbelievable. *Tea Tree Oil* is amazing. You can't take it internally or use it for more than two weeks for the sinuses. You can use it as a mouthwash to gargle with for your gums, but do not swallow it.

Various Infections

Yeast Infection

I have also had a yeast infection. When we have too much yeast in our body we can contract a yeast infection. Yeast infections are an overgrowth of yeast in the body. The doctors always recommend cream or vaginal suppositories and there are no side effects. I do the natural cure; I do not use the suppositories or any of the creams. I use my own formula which is water and an herb called **Bayberry** *Bark* tea. I boil the herbs in a pot of water, let it cool down and once it cools down, I use it as a douche. It makes me feel very clean from the inside. I like using this natural herb and it has no known side effects. Most yeast infections occur when we have too many sugary foods in our body and have worn tight underwear that prevents our body from breathing. If your underwear has dye and you do not wear panty liners to protect your skin from the dye, it can cause you to have this type of infection. *Bayberry Bark* is excellent for the yeast infections.

Respiratory Infection

I remember my husband was sneezing and coughing. After kissing my husband, all of a sudden we both have a pain in the chest and sneezing, coughing and we are spitting out phlegm. We both go to the doctor and the doctor diagnosed us with an upper respiratory infection. He gives us some antibiotics for the infection. Of course, I do not argue with them. I just take the prescription and as we go to the drugstore, I get my husband's prescription filled and I did not get my prescription filled.

My husband asked me,

"Why don't you want your prescription filled?"

I said, "No I am not taking that medicine because it has a lot of side effects, and you should not take it either."

My husband gives me a confused look, but he decided he was going to take his anyway. So we get home, I take my natural cures, my husband takes his medicine and we start the same day. My husband has taken his and I take my *Cat's Claw* and my *Devil's claw*. One is for inflammation; the other is to help you feel better for pain. They work very well together for whatever may be bothering you. I took the *Cat's claw* and the *Devil's claw* and I drank some organic flu medicine. Within a week I was better and my husband was still wheezing and sneezing and taking his medicine.

I laughed and teased him so much.

I said,

"Look at this, you took the doctors' medicine because you thought it was going to make you better faster then me. I took my natural medicine and I healed my body faster then you did with just natural herbs and I don't have any side effects."

To this day I still tease him about our bout with the upper respiratory infection. He could not believe I used natural medicine and within a week I was better.

It took my husband another week before he was better while taking the doctors medicine. It goes to show you that I am really into my natural herbs. All my herbs are always purchased from one store called the Merchants of the World Store, LLC. Their website is **www.Merchantsoftheworldstore.com** they have the best selection of herbs. They are 100% organic and they are really good and beneficial for my body. When I go into this shop, I get so excited I feel like a little kid in a candy store. I took courses in herbal medicine before I met the owners of *Merchants of the World Store, LLC.* This store has herbs that were hard to find in many stores. When I came upon this store I was so excited because I realized, all my prayers have been answered. This store has everything, including powders, pills, and herbal roots. What I mean by roots is that some herbs that are actually little roots of the plant. Some times we must use the root of the plant to make the tea or cream correctly. There is a wonderful plant (herb) called Blood Roots. This herb needs the root of the plant in order to make it a potent cream. However, you must be very careful and knowledgeable when using this herb because too much can be toxic.

Merchants is a wonderful store, and has a great website to place orders. The owners are wonderful people, and they are very knowledgeable of all the herbs and their different uses. **www.Merchantsoftheworldstore.com**

Boil on Buttocks Area

I go onto another little discomfort called a boil on my buttocks area. A boil is filled with pus and blood. A doctor would have to cut or lance it in order to get rid of it. They would have to squeeze the boil for the pus to drain out. I have never had one before now, but have heard women say it is very painful and uncomfortable. My mother had one and said it was very painful. Just my luck now I have a boil. My boil was in a very uncomfortable spot and it grew very large. One day I felt a little bump there, and wondered what it was. It hurts and is very tender, but I thought nothing about it. I figured it would go away it was just a bump. Everyday it was starting to grow, it was very large and it was painful. It was getting difficult to walk or sit. I did not know what was going on because I have never had one. When I told my mother, she said,

"Oh that is a boil and there is pus in there that needs to be drained before it gets too large."

By now you know my thoughts about conventional medicine.

She tells me you must go to the doctor to lance it and it is very painful. I did not want to go and have it cut.

At the same time this was happening, I was in school studying to become a certified holistic naturalist. I had class that day and was in a lot of pain, but I had to attend my class. I began to think, how am I going to do this? Before I left the house I had some herbs and I looked in my book and was informed to use *Cat's Claw* for the infection and *Blessed Thistle* for the female area. I got the *Blessed Thistle* and *Cat's Claw*; and proceeded to make a paste. I took a little vegetable oil and opened two capsules of both herbs to make a paste. I took that little paste that I made and put it on the affected area. I also put on a sanitary napkin for protection just in case something happens. When I made the paste (salve), I also took the capsules as well. At this point, I could barely walk. I had to drive 20 minutes to get to the class. Now imagine, if that wasn't bad enough, the class was all day. I had to be there from 9 am. to 5 pm. You can just imagine how excruciating that was for me. So I move very slowly and I get to class on time. While I am in class, the doctor, who is a naturalist, is talking and instructing us on natural herbs.

At this point, I had to excuse myself to visit the ladies room because I felt a little wetness. I went to the ladies room and I had to urinate. As I urinated the boil started to drain. Remember, I only used salve early that morning before I went to class. The salve made the boil come to a head or (burst), and when I looked down in the toilet I saw blood and pus from the boil. I was so excited and so happy, that it happened so quickly. I was amazed. I really did not think it would happen that fast because that was the first day I put the salve on it.

After looking in the toilet realizing how quickly the boil drained, I was elated to know I was in the right place taking classes to become a certified naturalist. This stuff was just too good to keep to myself. I must spread the word to others about the healing properties of God's natural herbs. It is just miraculous; I can't say enough about God's healing plants.

If you treat your body right with the right food and nourishment, and correct natural products you can be healed.

Chapter 12
Scoliosis (crooked spine)

Now, I have one more disease. I was born with
scoliosis and it is when the spine is curved. Most
spines are straight but sometimes people are born
with curved spines. Some curves can be very
deforming and painful, where others may be mild.
There are different degrees of the curvature of the
spine.

In the following pages I will give you thorough
information on Scoliosis and its minimal cures. In
some cases there is not much that can be done. I
have learned to live with this disease. Unfortunately,
my spine has a little more severe curve than most
people.

Scoliosis is a bending and twisting of the spinal
column affecting mainly the thoracic (middle spine)
or lumbar (lower spine). It is sometimes progressive
and distorts the chest and back. If left untreated, it
can lead to severe deformity.

The spine has an important role. The spine supports our erect posture, stabilizes our limbs relative to our trunks, supports our abdominal and thoracic regions, and protects our natural elements. The spine is in balance when the head is aligned with the pelvis. Scoliosis is a condition in which the spine is curved in the coronal or frontal plane. The coronal plane is the view from the crown (corona) of the head down. The frontal plane is the view of the body from the front. Scoliosis encompasses curves of 10 degrees and greater.

Besides physical deformity, it can lead to malfunctioning of organs that get misplaced and misaligned, causing problems of the respiratory, digestive, endocrine and other body systems. In rare, severe cases, scoliosis can lead to premature death.

A straight spine is essential for good health. It ensures that all the organs of the body are in their rightful places and that nerve signals are transmitted smoothly from the brain via the spinal cord to the rest of the body.

First, the spine does not develop its normal front to back arches, and this causes unusual weight to be carried on the spinal disc.

Second, the center of certain discs shifts to one side, and the vertebra tip to the other side, just like a teeter-totter. This misalignment, called a subluxation, causes the spine to tip to one side. To compensate for this bend, the spine then tips to the other side at another level and the result is scoliosis.

Possible Causes:

Scoliosis may be caused by a number of factors, including;

-abnormalities in the vertebra at birth

-regular and prolonged improper use of the body, such as carrying heavy loads on one side of the body;

-flat feet, uneven leg lengths and other conditions that cause a person to walk in an unbalanced manner;

-uneven stress or muscle tension, where the muscles on some parts of the body are perpetually more tense/tighter than other parts.

-other injuries to the developing spine.

Screening for scoliosis:

Often, family or friends first detect scoliosis in an adolescent by noticing an asymmetry in the shoulders, rib cage, waist, or pelvis. Screening is useful if early identification permits treatment that may halt the progression of the deformity. A simple test to recognize scoliosis is by bending over from the waist while keeping the legs and arms straight and the palms together. From the rear, a clear rib bulge will be visible if one has scoliosis. A common sign of the problem is one shoulder blade being more prominent than the other, with the tendency to lean a little to one side. The hips may be uneven. Most gym teachers, if you have physical education, will detect the problem early on.

Treatment Options:

Physical Therapy – A chiropractor is an excellent way to improve function, flexibility, endurance, and decrease pain. Usually the therapist will work with patients toward becoming less symptomatic, and maintaining the improvement with an active home exercise program. Working out in a supervised environment with the help of a physical therapist is the best way to achieve it. On average, therapy lasts 2-3 times per week for 4-8 weeks.

It is very important that adult patients with scoliosis get into the habit of doing a daily exercise routine.

This will improve the strength of the trunk muscles and take some of the stress off from the spine.

Often when pain occurs, it is because the patient is not doing his or her exercises.

Back Brace:

Is helpful in getting some relief from back pain in patients with degenerative scoliosis. When discovered at an early age, most doctors recommend using a back brace on children. When used in conjunction with the Scoliosis Treatment and Recovery System there can often times be up to a 50% or more correction over a period of 18- 36 months. Time depends on the range of curvature and compliance with the program. A word of caution is in order however: the brace should not be used without faithful compliance with an active exercise program. Brace wear without exercise tends to lead to a weaker spine that becomes dependent on the brace. Daily exercises and occasional (when needed) brace wear lead to the best results, where bracing is concerned.

Management of Scoliosis is determined by the:

-degree of the deformity

-location of the deformity

-cause of the deformity

-age of the patient

-skeletal maturity of the patient

-individual preferences of the patient and family.

According to medical science, there is "no cure" for scoliosis. The only medical treatment available is surgery to insert a metal rod into the spine, to force it straight. This is not an ideal solution, however, as it does not allow free movement of the individual vertebrae.

Now that I have given you a little history about scoliosis I will share my experience.

As I mentioned earlier I was born with this disease. My scoliosis was never detected as a child. I went through most of my life and school years, and never got a back brace to help correct the problem. My family and I did not know I had a twisted spine. However, there were signs of a problem. When I was a child I recall an incident with a gray coat that my grandmother brought me. It was a present to wear for church on Easter Sunday. I hated that coat, because my shoulders were uneven, therefore, the coat did not fit properly.

As I tried the coat on, I remember my grandmother asking my mom, "why is one shoulder higher than the other side." The coat did not fit right, because the one with the lower shoulder was so obviously different from the other. At the time in the 50's, the coats were designed with huge shoulder pads. Now just imagine huge uneven shoulder pads on a skinny nine-year-old child. The funny part is my grandmother kept trying to adjust the shoulders to no avail. Everyone assumed I had bad posture.

I do not blame my family for overlooking my problem. They were not taught about scoliosis or how to determine if your child had it. Somehow the doctors and my school missed my scoliosis. I was a little disappointed that the medical doctors never noticed my uneven shoulders or much higher hip. Fortunately, we got through it and I wore the coat.

As years went on, and I went through my adolescence stage, everything changed and I developed problems. At this time in my life, I did not know I had scoliosis and that all my organs were shifted out of proper alignment.

I had problems when I got my monthly periods. I remember my cramps were so bad they were unbearable. I would sleep on a cold hard floor; because that was the only place I found relief from the pain. I could not sleep in a bed; my mother could not understand why I was having such horrible cramps. She never experienced cramps like mine. My sisters who had their monthly periods, as well, never had cramps so severe. I was the only one that always had these excruciating cramps. It was so bad that I would get sick to my stomach and regurgitate. I could not go to school on those days. When I became an adult and started working, there were times I had to take days off from work because the pain was just that bad. I visited many doctors to no avail. My mom would take me to my visits and they would all say,

"It is okay, as soon as she has her first child, it will stop and she won't have these bad cramps anymore."

They gave me medication, and on the medicine was a special warning label indicating this medicine should be taken with strict precautions for a short time only.

I remember taking the medicine for the cramps, and I would be in so much pain and within minutes I would be on cloud nine. I would be in euphoria. I felt as if I could conquer the world. My whole demeanor would change and I was happy, just floating and wanting to sleep. My mom noticed the change when I took those pills, but she did not know exactly what was happening. My younger sister was attending a nursing high school. She happened to see the pills one day, and after reading the label she exclaimed,

"Oh! My goodness, Vivian do you know what this means?"

I answered, "No".

She said, "This is a warning these pills are addictive."

"How long have you been taking them?"

I said well,

"I only take them when I have bad cramps four days out of the month."

She said,

"You can't take this anymore, they are very addictive."

She told me to throw them out. I replied,

"I can't because they help me with my cramps." I thank God my sister noticed the pill before any damage was done. It was a miracle I did not become addicted but the truth was, I liked the way they made me feel and they got rid of my horrible cramps. When I took the pills, I could function like a normal person.   When the pills would get into my system, I would slow down nod off to sleep. I guess maybe that is why my mom did not really know what was happening to her oldest child. The sad part is I was getting high legally in the privacy of my own home at a young age. At this point I did not want to give up my pills, however, my sister insisted I had to and she told my mom. I gave up the pills, and that just goes to show you that I could have become addicted to prescription drugs at a young age.   When I think about it, I get upset with medical doctors. All the years I would constantly go to them and they never once gave me a simple spine test or checked my hips to see if they were   aligned evenly. Or never once checked my shoulders to notice that one side was higher than the other. Nor did they look at my hips to see that one side of my hip was much higher than the other. Never once thought to take an x-ray to see why she is having such bad cramps.   Instead they just gave me a month's supply of highly addictive medication. Unfortunately, if you are less fortunate and live in a certain neighborhood some things will be overlooked.

After having the menstrual problem, it got worse. As I got older I started to have digestive problems and my doctors would tell me,

"You are eating too late, do not eat this, and do not eat that."

I would tell the doctors when I try to swallow my food; it feels like a fist is trying to go down my esophagus. I can almost feel the food moving very slowly down my esophagus. Of course, they gave me more pills to take. I was also an extremely skinny person. I was the thinnest person in my family. My mom took me to the doctor to see why I could not gain weight. Due to my digestive problems I did not want to eat.

Remember, at this time I still am not aware that I have scoliosis and neither are the doctors.

Unfortunately, after the birth of my daughter due to my scoliosis, large fibroid, toxemia (Toxemia is pregnancy induced hypertension); and 50 pounds of weight gain all my body organs shifted. My organs were slightly shifted due to my curved spine, and having all these other changes made things worse. The changes wrecked havoc on my internal organs. I was unaware that my internal organs shifted. When I would eat, it would hurt so badly for me to try and swallow food. Literally, it felt like it would sit right on top of my chest and would not go down. Years later the chiropractor said my stomach was pushed up and in a tighter space due to my twisted spine.

I could not figure out what was wrong. I am not proud of what I had to resort to, but I would take my fingers and force myself to bring up my food. This went on for most of the time immediately after my baby's delivery. It went on so long that I became so accustomed to it that I did not have to force myself anymore. All I had to do was eat, wait a few minutes, go into the bathroom and bend over the toilet and everything would come up.

I could have become bulimic but I did not, and I thank God for that. I thank God that I have a strong constitution and that I did it out of necessary and pain. I realized it was becoming serious when I no longer had to force myself to throw up. I had lost control. I prayed and asked God to help me. I got some relief shortly after I lost most of the baby weight gain.

It is amazing how our loved ones can do things in privacy and no one is aware. After reading this book, all my friends and family will know all of my health struggles and victories.

After having my baby girl, I visited my doctor and I told him,

"Something is wrong, I do not know what is going on but my body is not right."

Of course, because I had a baby and my daughter was only a couple weeks old, the doctor could not find anything wrong. He attributed it to my gaining weight and having a fibroid. I listened and went home.

I started to lose my pregnancy weight by going to the gym and trying to get myself back together and the weight fell off. I did not have that much of a problem anymore with my digestive system because I would chew my food very slowly, and would eat a lot of soup.

Serious Back Pain

Many years later in my mid 40's, I was sitting at my office desk. I was an Administrative Assistant and would arrive to work at 8:00 in the morning. Most of the time I had lunch at my desk and I would not leave the office until 6 pm and sometimes later. Those were a lot of hours to sit. I noticed that my back was starting to hurt, but I did not complain I just dealt with it. One day I got up to get dressed for work and I could barely put on my clothes. My back was stiff, however, I went to work anyway. Later that day I could not get up from my desk, my back locked on me. It was really bad and I went to the company nurse. I told the nurse that there was something wrong with my back, and do not send me to a medical doctor they can not help me, something is seriously wrong.

The nurse said,

"You workout every day, you are on the treadmill, you jog, you probably pulled a muscle or something."

I said, "No, I do not think so."

"Please send me to a chiropractor."

I can't go to a medical doctor. She sent me to a chiropractor she recently met at a health conference two days before I went to her office. He was definitely sent by God because he was a great doctor. Anyway, I went to the chiropractor and on the first visit, he tells me,

"Ms., what have you been experiencing with your back?"

I told him my problem.

He said,

"I am going to take an x-ray of your back. Come back in two days I should have the x-ray, and we will discuss the results."

He said,

"I can't tell you what is wrong. I do not know your history, and can't give you any advice until I look at your x-ray."

He did get to tell me how the vertebrae and spine works. I found it to be very interesting. I went back to his office two days later. While I am in his office he has another patient, and he tells me to go into one of his rooms and put on a top robe. I changed into the little shirt they gave me and I waited. I am looking at the photos that he has of the vertebrae, and then my eye catches this x-ray. I see this x-ray and I thought to myself,

"That x-ray looks like it belongs to a 90-year-old. The spine looks like the letter **S**, I would hate to be that person."

The doctor comes into the office and he says to me,

"Vivian, I got your x-ray back, I do not know your medical history and we have never met before, right."

I said, "Right."

He said, "I know nothing about your life."

I said, "Right."

He said,

"From your x-ray, I know your whole life's story."

He said,

"You should have one side of your shoulder much higher than the other, and one hip should be much higher than the other. You should have a problem with your heel on your left foot. He said, it should have bothered you and you should have worn out your shoes on that side much quicker than the other."

 He also said,

"You should have had very bad digestive problems; and you should have excruciating monthly periods."

When he told me that I cried like a baby. Just thinking about it right now brings tears to my eyes again. This man, who never knew me, never met me, took one look at my x-ray and told me my *whole life's story*. All the pain and suffering that I had for years. I am a middle-aged woman in his office, and for the first time in my life I hear the words,

"**You have scoliosis!**"

I did not know what scoliosis was.

Then he said to me,

"You see that x-ray right up there,"

I said, "Yes",

He said, "That is your spine."

When he told me that I wanted to pass out. I could not believe that was my spine no way, how could this go undetected for so many years, how? What happened, why were the doctors so negligent in giving me an x-ray exam? That is all it would have taken. Even the chiropractor said,

"Vivian, I can't believe that you went to a school where they were supposed to check you for this. You went to the doctors and nobody gave you an x-ray of the spine."

He implied,

"The doctors only gave you that addictive medication for your pain."

He explained the reason I was having horrible cramps is because my spine was curved and it was touching major organs including my stomach. My pelvic was tilted and when my ovaries swelled each month, there was no room for them to enlarge to release the eggs that were not fertilized. He said, due to the birth of my daughter, the esophagus and stomach area had shifted causing my horrible indigestion problems.

He indicated,

"All they had to do was take an x-ray."

From that day on I was out of work for three months with back problems. I could not go to work because I could not sit, and I could not even walk that is how bad it was. I had to lie on my floor most of the time for three months. I could barely sit, I could barely stand, and I could barely walk it was really bad, my back was really, really bad. My doctor informed me that I could no longer work at my present position anymore. I could end up in a wheelchair he warned and said,

"The hours are too long and you must change your position. You make the choice!"

He wrote a note to my supervisor and my boss stating I could no longer sit for that long. Of course, they made changes to accommodate me. My hours had to be the normal 9 am – 5 pm. Not from 9 am to 6 pm or later. It had to be normal work hours, and I had to take a break every couple of minutes to leave my desk and stretch my back. My job was very hectic and required many hours of sitting at my desk. I could not leave my desk for fear that an important client would call and I would not be available to take the call. So we had to make some changes at work and within three months the doctor had me back on my feet.

He had to manipulate my back. Manipulation is actually when he tries to force my spine to straighten up a little. Because of my age I was too old to wear a back brace. I went to the orthopedic doctor for the spine and he suggested I put two metal rods in my back.

My reply was,

"You are out of your mind! At my age I am not going to put two metal rods in my back, no way."

I went back to my chiropractor and he would manipulate the vertebrae. He would press down on them and when he pressed they moved. When they moved you could hear a cracking sound. It was weird the first time, but after going there three times out of the week I got used to the sound. He had to teach me how to walk all over again, and how to properly sit to allow support of my spine. He taught me how to Stretch, bend from my knees, bend over and how to lift things.

Also, I learned how to walk with my head up to elongate my neck and my body. It was a lot of work but amazingly, after three months I was back at work doing well. My life changed completely.

I know there are certain things that I can't do. I have to sit a certain way and can't sit too long, because I still have scoliosis. There is nothing I can do about it and there is nothing they can do.

I still visit the chiropractor frequently. I go to a chiropractor maybe 10 times a year. I go for maintenance and that is to adjust my spine and get it back where it needs to be. Sometimes I may need more treatment depending on if I am experiencing back pain. My scoliosis starts from the middle of my neck and it goes down my back. I have to be very careful with my spine and what I do. My chiropractor told me that God built the body to heal itself naturally. The spine is the nucleus of the body and all the nerves go from the vertebrates. Hand manipulation is all it takes to heal the body naturally. He said,

"I do not believe in any medicine, I will not give you any pills; I will not prescribe anything. We are naturalists and we will just work with the hands."

Sure enough he worked with his hands and within three months I was back to normal without medication. People tell me you believe in the quacks. They are not quacks for me because the medical doctors could not do anything for me. For years they did not find anything wrong with me. They gave me medicine but they never once took a simple x-ray that could have solved all my problems. From that day forward I believed in chiropractors. The chiropractor was the first experience I had with a naturalist doctor, and going to the chiropractor was a rude awakening for me.

Just a note: *As of the writing of this book, I am praying and believing through Jesus (Yeshua) he will supernaturally straighten my spine. The bible states, "...if you have the faith of a mustard seed you can say to the mountain move, and it will move"... (KJB) Matt: 17:20.*

Once the doctor talked about natural healing, and how the body naturally heals itself, is when I really got interested in natural healing. Even though I had already dabbled a little bit in the herbs in my 20s, the biggest part came from the chiropractor. He opened my mind up to natural healing and I was a great candidate because I was in a lot of pain. I saw what he could do and what the medical doctors could not do.

Due to my condition, I will always have to exercise and walk. It keeps my back strong. My posture is somewhat bad due to the curved spine. I will always have a problem with indigestion, if my weight increases, because my stomach is shifted out of its proper alignment. I must wear a special shoe insert support for my left foot. It is to accommodate for the shorter leg. Sometimes when I walk without the support, my left foot gets very painful. However, through it all I am grateful because it could be worse. I make the best of every day.

My very good friend's son was complaining about back pain. He was only ten years old. She took him to an Orthopedic Doctor. He discovered her son's feet were hurting because he had extremely flat feet. He had no arch support at all and it gave him back problems. The doctor made supports for his feet and the pain immediately ceased.

Parents please pay attention to your children's back and especially when they complain of back pain. It only takes a minute to see a doctor, but a lifetime of pain if it goes uncorrected. I hate to sound bias but I know there are some things that medical doctors have to do. I love medical doctors as well. I go to them constantly and get my diagnosis. Please do not make the mistake of not seeing and getting a diagnosis from your medical doctor before you take herbs. There comes a point when you may have to get an operation for whatever reason. However, I still love my naturalist doctors. My doctors were great and I am grateful. I am thankful to God that I had these experiences. Due to my experiences, what I have been through, I pray that I may help other people when they hear my story. I have told them what to do, what to use, where to go. I thank God because I have been through it. I am not telling you what I have heard, what someone has told me, or what I have seen. I am actually a living witness, a living testimony. What I had, how we worked it, how it cleared up, just by using God's natural healing plants what he put here for man.

". . . by the waters . . . will be trees the fruit will be your food and the leaves will be your medicine." (KJV) Ezekiel 47:12

Even then in the biblical days God thought of everything in our natural medicine. I am so thankful that I have had this journey with the herbs; and that I can tell other people about my journey. Hopefully, they will have as much success with the herbs and the natural healing of the body as I have had.

As I publish this book in paperback form, I am elated to say through prayer and faith my **Scoliosis** is healed. Your probably thinking well how can that be? With faith and prayer all things are possible.

"...by his stripes we are healed." Isaiah 53:5
"...I am the God that healeth thee." Exodus 15:26

Chapter 13
Iridology

There is another aspect of natural healing I would like to mention, and that is the art of Iridology. I have a good friend who is a Naturalist Doctor, M.D. and also specializes in Iridology.

What is Iridology? An **alternative medicine** technique whose proponents believe those patterns, colors, and other characteristics of the *iris* can be examined to determine information about a patient's health. Practitioners match their observations to *iris charts*, which divide the iris into zones that correspond to specific parts of the human body. Iridologists see the eyes as "windows" into the body's state of health.

Iridologists use the charts to distinguish between healthy systems and organs in the body and those that are overactive, inflamed, or distressed. Iridologists believe this information demonstrates a patient's susceptibility towards certain illnesses, reflects past medical problems, or predicts later health problems.

That colored part of your eye is not just color. It is made up of thousands of nerve fibers. Approximately twenty eight thousand individual nerve fibers to be exact. When you look closely at your own eye, what looks like individual fibers, are actually a cable of fibers made up of about twelve to twenty-five nerve fibers wrapped together.

These nerve fibers come from every part of your body from your skin down to your bones. These nerve fibers then travel up your spinal cord to your brain (hypothalamus) then to your iris (via the ophthalmic branch of the trigeminal ganglion). These fibers change in reflex to the change of nerve energy in any affiliated area of the body.

Now, getting back to my friend the doctor. I remember the first time meeting her. We were both at an herbal holistic workshop. She introduced herself to me and informed me what her profession was. She then proceeded to look into my eyes and give me my history.

She said,

"This is my first time meeting you, but I can see from your iris that you were in a car accident, and not just one but two car accidents; and you have a mild heart problem."

I was absolutely flabbergasted, because I never believed in iridology; and my heart was fine as far as I knew. I actually took offense to that because I did not want to believe something was wrong with my heart. However, she was right I was in two minor car accidents. She got the car accidents correct, and there was absolutely no way she could have known that. For goodness sake, I just met these people for the first time and no one knew my past. However, she proved me wrong. She indicated Iridology was her specialty.

Now, fast forwarding one year later. I am getting my annual check up and my doctor gave me an EKG, and it came back abnormal. He takes it again, and again it is abnormal. At this time, I am feeling great and I have no idea what the doctor is talking about. Now I go to the cardiologist again. Since the doctors found a problem, I am now feeling a little rapid heart beat. Nothing serious, just a rapid heart beat most likely from pre-menopause symptoms. They suggested medicine or a procedure to correct the problem. Of course, I rejected the procedure and medicine.

You see, the Iridologist saw the problem before I did. Since that incident we have become good friends and she is doing well with her practice; and I have taken a small course to study the Iris. Don't get me wrong; to become an expert like my friend she had to take many extensive courses studying the Iris. She told me all her medical training consisted of 12 years and she has many degrees to prove it.

Again, there are many excellent doctors. I would never put my health at risk, I get my annual check ups every year. Medical doctors are a very important aspect of our lives. Not everyone believes in the natural healing and that is why God gave the medical doctors their desire and knowledge to heal people. Everyone is different, you be the judge, you decide whether you want natural healing or conventional.

I would like to mention that the best way to avoid getting sick is by eating a healthy diet and regular exercising. I can't stress that enough. Eat less fast food; take time to make fresh home cooked meals. If you must eat out, go to a nice sit down restaurant where you know they cook fresh. Eat less sugar, white breads, and starches, red meat and pork. It is never too late to start a healthy diet. At one of my health workshop, I had people ask me,

"Is it expensive to buy organic foods?"

My reply,

"You will either pay for it now to eat healthy or pay for it later in life by hospital stays and expensive medicine. You make the choice. You are what you eat, *"junk in, junk out."*

Some people think we can eat anything we want and take a magic pill, whether it is herbal or conventional medicine and the problem will go away. The problem does not go away; the medicine just masks the problem. As soon as you stop taking the medicine the problem is back with a vengeance. The best prevention is to eat healthy and exercise.

I know for a fact, there are many people that take all types of conventional medication for diabetes, high blood pressure, high cholesterol but eat everything the doctor tells them is causing these problems. However, they continue to eat all the bad food and pop a pill only to wake up another day and repeat their same bad behavior.

**Just a Note: If you want to get the most beneficial health results, you must be consistent in your diet and medicine be it conventional or herbal.

"LET YOUR FOOD BE YOUR MEDICINE AND YOUR MEDICINE BE YOUR FOOD." By *Hippocrates*

Chapter 14
Various Herbs

Below is a list of the various herbs mentioned in this book which I have used:

Herbs

Red Clover: Possible Benefits:
- Helps prevent cancer, tumors
- Used to treat menopausal symptoms
- Good for skin inflammations
- Relaxes the body
- Has Isoflavones to help reduce hot flashes and prevent osteoporosis
- Fights infection
- Suppresses appetite and purifies the blood
- Good for eczema
- Blood thinner

Nutrient Content:
Calcium, iron, magnesium, manganese, phosphorus, potassium, selenium zinc, vitamins B_3, C, and E.

Caution: should not be used with any other blood thinners. First week of taking may make you a little constipated until your body adjusts.

Garlic: Possible Benefits:
- Lowers blood pressure
- Improves circulation
- Helps stabilize blood lipid levels
- Great for colds and flu
- Dissolves plaque in arteries
- Circulatory problems
- Lowers cholesterol levels

Caution: Has blood thinning properties do not use with other blood thinners

Nutrient Content:
Calcium, folate,iron, magnesium, manganese, phosphorus, potassium selenium, zinc, vitamins B_1, B_2, B_3, and C.

Tea Tree Oil: Possible Benefits: ·
- Used topically
- Disinfects wounds and heals virtually all skin conditions
- Acne, Athlete's foot, cuts, burns
- Infections, hair and scalp problems
- Herpes outbreaks, insect a bites
- Vaginitis
- Gargle for colds
- Mouth sores
- Sore throats
- Sinuses

Caution: Should not be taken internally or swallowed, it can be toxic.

Nutrient Content:
Oil

Bayberry Bark: Possible Benefits:
- Decongestant and astringent
- Aids circulation
- Immune system
- Vaginal Douche
- Fever

Caution: Should not be used at high dosages or for prolonged periods. May irritate sensitive stomachs.

Nutrient Content:
Calcium, iron, magnesium, manganese, phosphorus, potassium, selenium, silicon, zinc, vitamins B_1, B_3 and C.

Cats Claw: Possible Benefits:
- Antioxidant
- Anti-inflammatory
- Helps immune system
- Viral infections
- Arthritis
- Cancer
- Tumors
- Ulcers

Caution: Should not be used during pregnancy

Nutrient Contents:
Mitraphyline, oleanolic acid, pteropodine, ursolic acid

Devils Claw: Possible Benefits:
- Relieves Pain
- Reduces inflammation
- Acts as a diuretic
- Sedative
- Great for back pain
- Arthritis, rheumatism, diabetes
- Allergies
- Liver
- Gallbladder

Caution: Should not be used during pregnancy or nursing.

Nutrient Content:
Calcium, iron, magnesium, manganese, phosphorus, potassium, selenium, zinc

Blessed Thistle: Possible Benefits:
- Stimulates the appetite
- Heals the liver
- Anti-inflammation
- Improves circulation
- Good for female disorders
- Cleanses the blood
- Strengthens the heart
- Increases milk flow in nursing mothers

Caution: none

Nutrient Content:
Calcium, essential fatty acids, iron, magnesium, manganese, phosphorus, potassium, selenium, silicon, zinc, vitamins B_1, B_2, B_3, and C

CAUTION: BEFORE TAKING ANY TYPE OF HERBS OR MEDICINE ALWAYS CONSULT WITH YOUR DOCTOR. DO NOT TAKE HERBS IF PREGNANT OR NURSING.

Conclusion

What really amazes me is that I have been through so much physically in my life and I am sure so have many others. However, I did not let my situations get me down. The situations just made me work harder to be as healthy as I can be. I am 60 years old and feel like 25 and I don't look or feel my age. Many people have asked me if my hair is natural, and yes it is my natural hair. At my age most people lose their hair, but my hair is getting longer and thicker. I do not use products to grow my hair it just grows naturally. I am retired and ready to start a new career, and seek greater endeavors. I have much to live for and much to give. I am not ready for the rocking chair because I have too much energy. I am a baby boomer and many of my friends and family are sick or dead, because of their bad eating habits and lack of exercise. So many of them are unwilling to go the distance and take back their lives. Most diseases can be reversed with proper diet and exercise. I did not let the doctors' diagnosis limit me to a life of sickness. I walk by Faith and not sight. I believed in God's natural healing plants and I used them to the fullest. I thank God everyday for his healing plants and using me as a *living testimony* for others. You too can have health and energy if you choose to make the decision.

We must get healthier and take charge of our health!

When shopping, purchase meats that say "all natural" or "no hormones used". They cost a little more, but it's worth it. By eating hormone free meat, this should prevent the fibroids from regrowing.

Again, **LET YOUR FOOD BE YOUR MEDICINE AND YOUR MEDICINE BE YOUR FOOD.**

I thank you. I wish you well and may God bless you.

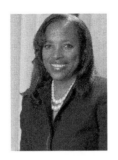

ABOUT THE AUTHOR

Vivian Moody Perry is happily married with one daughter.

She is a Certified Naturalist Consultant and used natural herbs to heal herself. Vivian has not used conventional medicine for many years. However, she had some ailments which doctors have claimed that she most likely was born with. If you read her story, you will find out about all of the "diseases" that she has endured, and how with God's natural healing plants (herbs) she was healed.

She loves to do humanitarian work and is the Founder and President of her family's non-profit Childrens' Foundation, the "Vincent Moody Foundation." They provide clothing and toys for the homeless. She enjoys conducting health workshops and empowering people to be the best they can be.

Her goal and mission is to continue to help the homeless; and acquire homes to shelter the young adults that have aged out of Foster Care and have nowhere to live.

Please check out my latest health workshop videos.

Remember to keep in touch and visit my websites and You tube Channel (www.youtube.com/shrink fibroids and Facebook Fan Page, Vivian Moody Perry "How to Shrink Fibroids") for new updates.

www.HealthyHerbforFibroids.com
www.VivianMoodyPerry.com
email: vivianmoodyperry@gmail.com

aqua Panna
Pellegrino

Made in the USA
Lexington, KY
31 January 2013